Chidambaram Sivamani Rajmohan
G. Sivagami
D. Sendhilnathan

Measurement of pulpal temperature while using resin luting cements

AF135583

Chidambaram Sivamani Rajmohan
G. Sivagami
D. Sendhilnathan

Measurement of pulpal temperature while using resin luting cements

Temperature rise caused while luting ceramic restoration with various resin cements, bonding agents and light sources

LAP LAMBERT Academic Publishing

Impressum / Imprint

Bibliografische Information der Deutschen Nationalbibliothek: Die Deutsche Nationalbibliothek verzeichnet diese Publikation in der Deutschen Nationalbibliografie; detaillierte bibliografische Daten sind im Internet über http://dnb.d-nb.de abrufbar.
Alle in diesem Buch genannten Marken und Produktnamen unterliegen warenzeichen-, marken- oder patentrechtlichem Schutz bzw. sind Warenzeichen oder eingetragene Warenzeichen der jeweiligen Inhaber. Die Wiedergabe von Marken, Produktnamen, Gebrauchsnamen, Handelsnamen, Warenbezeichnungen u.s.w. in diesem Werk berechtigt auch ohne besondere Kennzeichnung nicht zu der Annahme, dass solche Namen im Sinne der Warenzeichen- und Markenschutzgesetzgebung als frei zu betrachten wären und daher von jedermann benutzt werden dürften.

Bibliographic information published by the Deutsche Nationalbibliothek: The Deutsche Nationalbibliothek lists this publication in the Deutsche Nationalbibliografie; detailed bibliographic data are available in the Internet at http://dnb.d-nb.de.
Any brand names and product names mentioned in this book are subject to trademark, brand or patent protection and are trademarks or registered trademarks of their respective holders. The use of brand names, product names, common names, trade names, product descriptions etc. even without a particular marking in this works is in no way to be construed to mean that such names may be regarded as unrestricted in respect of trademark and brand protection legislation and could thus be used by anyone.

Coverbild / Cover image: www.ingimage.com

Verlag / Publisher:
LAP LAMBERT Academic Publishing
ist ein Imprint der / is a trademark of
OmniScriptum GmbH & Co. KG
Heinrich-Böcking-Str. 6-8, 66121 Saarbrücken, Deutschland / Germany
Email: info@lap-publishing.com

Herstellung: siehe letzte Seite /
Printed at: see last page
ISBN: 978-3-659-44349-7

Zugl. / Approved by: Chennai, The Tamil Nadu Dr. M.G.R. Medical University, Diss., 2006

Copyright © 2013 OmniScriptum GmbH & Co. KG
Alle Rechte vorbehalten. / All rights reserved. Saarbrücken 2013

CONTENTS

LIST OF FIGURES

LIST OF TABLES

ABSTRACT

Purpose of the study

The clinician should know whether the temperature rise caused while curing the dual cure resin cements and its bonding agents on the tooth prepared for all ceramic restorations that lacks sufficient remaining dentin thickness is harmful to the pulp or not.

Objectives

➢ To compare the temperature rise caused by different light curing sources used for curing one bonding agent.

➢ To compare the temperature rise using single light curing source used for curing different bonding agents.

➢ To compare the temperature rise caused by different light curing sources used for curing one resin cement.

➢ To compare the temperature rise using single light curing source used for curing different resin cements.

Materials and methods

Two coats of bonding agent were applied over the dentin disk and cured for 10 seconds using the high intensity halogen. The temperature change was recorded for every five seconds up to two minutes . The dual cure resin cement was mixed and placed inside the 10mm diameter, 0.75mm thick steel mold kept over the dentin disk. The ceramic disk was placed over this assembly and cured for 40 seconds. The temperature change was recorded for every five seconds up to two minutes. The experiment was repeated with different bonding agents and its corresponding dual cure resin cements with various light sources. In each group the experiment was repeated ten times. The difference in temperature rise from the initial to highest temperature was calculated for each sample (ΔT). The obtained readings (ΔT) were averaged for each group to determine the mean temperature rise for that particular group. The data's were tabulated and statistically analyzed using student's t-test, one way Anova and Tukey HSD.

Results

➢ When curing bonding agents LED (Satelec) produced the highest temperature rise

➢ When curing resin cements High intensity halogen produced the highest temperature rise

Conclusion

➢ Light sources have a significant influence on the rise of temperature during the curing of bonding agents and their corresponding dual cure resin cements.

➢ Choice of bonding agent and resin cement does not cause a statistically significant difference in the temperature rise with the single light source.

➢ The choice of LED's (Mectron and Satelec) affects the temperature rise when curing the luting cements.

➢ Sufficient time interval should be given between curing of bonding agents and curing of their corresponding resin cements.

➢ The rise of temperature in all the groups may not affect the pulpal health as they were well within the critical temperature of 5.5°C.

Keywords:- Temperature rise, Light curing unit, Dual cure resin cement, Bonding agent.

1. INTRODUCTION

The desire for tooth colour restorations has moulded the evolution of aesthetic dentistry to its present challenging, but promising form. Presently, ceramics are the material of choice for aesthetic restorations for their ability to reproduce the natural tooth texture, colour and translucency and also have proven to be stable and strong for a longer duration which enhances the functional requirements of intraoral restorations. The life of these restorations in the oral environment depends heavily on the quality of the luting agents used to cement them on the abutment teeth. At present, dual cure resin cements are recommended for ceramic restorations[1], which get polymerized by both chemical and visible light at wavelengths of 400 – 500nm.

The various light curing units [LCU] available are halogen lights, solid-state light emitting diodes [LED], lasers and plasma arc lamp. Among these units, halogen lights and LEDs are used widely. Halogen bulbs produce light when electric energy heats a small tungsten filament to high temperatures. It operates at light intensities between 400 and 800 mW/cm^2 and polymerize resin composite material within 40 seconds. Despite their common use in dentistry they have several disadvantages. The basic principle of light conversion by this technique is claimed to be inefficient, as the light power output is less than 1% of the consumed electric power, and such bulbs have a limited effective lifetime of approximately 100 hours because of degradation of bulb components by the high heat generated[2].

Light emitting diode was proposed in 1995 for the polymerization of light cured dental materials to overcome the shortcomings of halogen visible light curing agents[3]. Since its introduction into the market, LED light curing units have evolved considerably, especially in terms of irradiance. The first-generation LED LCUs presented an irradiance of 400 mW/cm^2 and a power output of 1 W. The second generation reached 800 mW/cm^2 and 5 W, and the third generation, which emerged recently, exceeds 1100 mW/cm^2 and 8 W. LEDs use doped semiconductor junctions (p-n junctions) to generate and emit light[4]. Under proper forward biased conditions, the injected electrons and holes recombine at a p-n junction and thereby emit light; in the case of gallium nitride LEDs, blue light is emitted. Additionally, a small polymer lens is included in front of the p-n junction to produce a partially collimated light[5-7]. The wavelength of light emitted by LEDs closely matches the absorption spectrum of camphoroquinone (CQ), a photoinitiator widely used in light-activated dental resins [3,5,6,8-10].

The advantages of LEDs [11] include: (1) narrow spectrum eliminates the light filter system required by other technologies, (2) efficiently converts electricity into light with less heat generation, and subsequently less cooling is required, (3) long service life as it routinely functions on battery- charging cycles and battery life, and (4) little or no degradation over time as compared to the degradation of lamp, filter, and reflector with time in conventional halogen units. Further, it has been recently demonstrated that blue GaN LED has the potential to cure composite resins to the effect of exceeding the minimum requirements of ISO standards for depth of cure and tensile strength.[6.] In view of the favorable results obtained, its performance can be considered clinically satisfactory.[12-14.]

Polymerization of dual cure resin cements results in a temperature increase caused by both exothermic reaction process of the material and light delivered from the curing unit[15-19]. The light cure units are capable of creating a temperature increase of up to 12°C[19]. This temperature rise has been shown to be a major source of heat that may damage the pulp[17].

These factors along with reduced remaining dentin thickness as seen in preparations for all ceramic restorations, produces a deleterious effect on the health of the pulp.

The lesser heat production of LEDs during routine and extended use of polymerization of light cured resin cements had been proved by Yap and Soh[20] and others[4,21-24]. Literature lacks information on the temperature rise in the pulp caused by LEDs while curing the dual cure resin cements and its bonding agents on the tooth prepared for all ceramic restorations that lacks sufficient remaining dentin thickness.

Hence the present in vitro study was designed with the following objectives:

➢ To compare the temperature rise in the pulp chamber caused by different light curing sources used for curing one bonding agent.

➢ To compare the temperature rise in the pulp chamber using single light curing source used for curing different bonding agents.

➢ To compare the temperature rise in the pulp chamber caused by different light curing sources used for curing one resin cement.

➢ To compare the temperature rise in the pulp chamber using single light curing source used for curing different resin cements.

2. REVIEW OF LITERATURE

Zach L and Cohen G[25] had done a study to find the effects of an externally applied known heat source on the pulp and the response was measured histologically. The Macaca rhesus monkey was selected as an experimental animal and the soldering iron tip was used to apply the heat on the external surface. The contact was maintained for periods of 5 to 20 seconds to produce an intrapulpal temperature increase of 4 -30°F. Specimens were obtained at intervals of 2, 7, 14, 56 and 91 days after heat application for histological evaluation. The results showed that there was no damage to the pulp when the temperature rise was within 4°F. But 15% and 60% of the teeth failed to recover when the temperature rise was 10°F and 20°F respectively. When the rise was 30°F all the teeth failed to recover. Hence it was concluded that, when all the operative procedures were carried out within 0–10°F the pulp was in the safe zone of recovery.

Tjan AHL and Dunn JR[26] had conducted a study in which they measured the temperatures of seven brands of visible light generators (Coelite, Elipar insight II with filter, insight II without filter, Translux, Visar 2 and Visilux II) at the light emitting tip of the light curing rod beneath a 1mm thick dentin disk and beneath a 2mm thick dentin disk during a 60 sec curing cycle. The temperature measurement was done on a mounted tooth sample submerged in a water bath (37°C) to standardize the surrounding temperature. The temperature was recorded at 5 seconds intervals for duration of 60 seconds irradiation. The process was verified three times at each of three levels for each light generator tested. The results of this study were

> Temperature rise was different for various tested light curing units. In all three locations of probe placement; the Translux unit produced the least temperature elevation.

> Thickness of residual dentin was a critical factor in reducing thermal transfer to the pulp.

Barghi N, Berry T and Hatton C[27] had examined the various curing units used in private practice offices to determine the adequacy of the units and related their output to various factors that might affect the intensity of the light produced by each unit. Radiometer was used to measure the light intensity and the dentists were interviewed to elicit information about the age of the unit. They concluded that

> About 30% of the units had an output of less than 200 mW/cm^2 which was inadequate to provide the desired degree of polymerization.

> Many dentists were unaware that the output of their curing light was inadequate for office use.

> The intensity of the light was inversely proportional to the age of the unit.

Shortall AC and Harrington E[28] compared the temperature rise produced by two light curing units of different output intensities at different distances - between the sensor and the light guiding tip (0mm, 2mm, 4mm, and 6mm). They also measured the temperature rise at the base of 2mm thick increments of 3 light activated posterior composite resin restoratives with two different opacities. They concluded that the temperature rise at the base of the cavity relates to

> Light transmission characteristics of resin composite

➤ Radiant energy output from the light curing unit.

➤ Polymerization exothermic of the material.

Hanning M and Bott B[29] had done a study that compared the in vitro pulp chamber temperature changes induced by a conventional halogen incandescent light source (Heliolux II) with those induced by 5 current visible light curing units (Astralis 5,ADT 1000 PAC system, Elipar highlight, Optilux 500,QHL 75) while curing a 2mm layer of composite in a class II cavity prepared in a lower third molar that had a RDT between pulp chamber and axial wall of the proximal box and pulp chamber and the occlusal cavity floor as 1mm. Measurements of the pulp chamber temperature changes during polymerization were performed with a K-type thermocouple placed at the pulp dentin junction. From this study it was concluded that the curing unit with high energy output (ADT 1000 PAC system) caused significantly higher pulp temperature changes as compared to the conventional curing unit.

Cobb DS et al[30] compared the temperature induced at the dentin-pulpal interface between the argon laser and the visible light curing unit at a variety of exposure regimens and conditions. The specimens used were human third molars that were sectioned exposing the pulp chamber. They were then filled with plastibase and the temperature changes were detected by a thermocouple.

The exposure regimens were

➤ Exposure of the tooth to light source with 1 mm intact dentin disk placed over the plastibase filled pulp chamber with continuous and interrupted cycles.

➤ Addition of 1 mm dentin disk placed on the top of the base disk and exposure through the disk.

➢ Exposure to the light source after placing a hole of 3 mm in diameter at the center of the upper disk.

➢ Exposure to the light source after placing composite in this hole.

➢ Final exposure after placing 2mm of base dentin disk.

It was concluded from this study that the argon laser consistently caused a smaller maximal temperature rise than did the Visible Light Curing unit and the thickness of dentin disk was inversely proportional to the temperature rise. The continuous exposure to both light sources produced higher temperature increase than did similar exposure times by using the interrupted cycle.

Porko C and Hietala EL[31] had done an in vitro study to explore the effect of light curing on the pulpal temperature. Ten extracted human molars were used in this study. The occlusal surfaces of these teeth were exposed to five consecutive 40 seconds light curing exposures and the temperature rise was measured immediately after each exposure with a thermocouple. The range of maximal temperature difference was 2.2°C. These teeth were again preserved totally under water until an occlusal cavity was prepared. A standard occlusal cavity was prepared in all the ten teeth and restored with etching, bonding and composite restoration. The adhesive was cured for 20 seconds and each increment of composite was cured for 40 seconds. An additional 40 seconds curing was done to ensure complete polymerization and the reading for temperature rise was measured with thermocouple. The range of maximal temperature difference was 7.2°C. Hence to conclude, the warming effect of pulp should be taken into account when curing large restorations that need several consecutive light curing exposures.

Loney RW and Price RBT[32] determined the effect of a concentrating light guide on a quartz tungsten halogen light curing unit and a plasma arc unit on the thermal transfer through resin and two different thickness of dentin. Two curing light sources used in this study were Optilux 401 with a standard 8mm light guide tip or a light concentrating tip and a plasma arc lamp (Apollo 95 E). Output of the Optilux curing light was measured prior to the experiment for the standard light guide (Optilux standard) and concentrating light guide (Optilux turbo) with and without an intervening mylar strip. The light output of the plasma arc unit could not be measured because it was beyond the upper limit of the light output measuring devices. Temperatures were directly measured at the tip of the light guide and through a combined sandwich of a precured cylinder of resin composite (1mm thick) and a cylindrical specimen of dentin (thin-0.58mm, thick-1.45mm). Temperatures were measured using thermocouple that was in direct contact with either the mylar strip or the surfaces of the dentin furthest away from the light guiding tip. The results of the study showed that the greatest temperature changes occurred when measured directly on the light guide of the curing light through the mylar strip. The temperature increase was lowest when measured through the 1mm composite and the 1.45 mm dentin sandwich. When measured through the combined composite/ dentin sandwich, the plasma arc unit, used for three seconds, produced the lowest temperature increase. For a given resin thickness, measured temperature changes were greatest for Optilux turbo and least for Apollo 95E. The temperature increased by 42% to 56% when the turbo light guide was used compared to the standard light guide used for thick and thin dentin specimens.

Knezevic A et al[33] compared the degree of conversion and temperature rise of four hybrid composite materials after illumination with two standard halogen curing units and blue superbrite LEDs on the surface of the composite materials and at 1mm depth. The degree of conversion was only little higher and the temperature rise was double with halogen light source when compared with LED. The temperature and degree of conversion obtained were higher on the surface than on 1mm depth regardless of the light source used. It was concluded that the LEDs with minimal intensity produced lower temperature rise and comparable degree of conversion when compared to halogen lights.

Yap AUJ and Sob MS[20] conducted a study to quantify and compare the thermal emission of three LEDs and halogen lights. Thermal emission of the light curing units when used in various curing modes were assessed using a K-type thermocouple and a digital thermometer at a distance of 3mm and 6mm and compared to the conventional halogen light curing unit. At 3mm the temperature rise ranged from 4.1°C to 12.9°C with LED light and 17.4°C to 46.4°C for halogen light. At 6 mm the temperature rise ranged from 2.4°C to 7.5°C for LED light and 7°C to 25.5°C for halogen light. They concluded that

> ➤ LED lights emit significantly less heat than the halogen lights.

> ➤ The heat emitted by individual curing light depends on the curing mode used.

> ➤ The heat emitted by different LED / halogen lights varies significantly.

Usumez A and Ozturk N[34] had done a study to measure the temperature increase induced by selected curing units - conventional halogen, high intensity halogen, plasma arc light and light emitting diode during resin cement polymerization under ceramic restoration. A ceramic specimen of 5 mm diameter and 2mm thickness (1mm thickness of framework material and 1mm thickness of layering material) and a dentin disk of 5mm diameter and 1mm height were prepared. Commercially available dual cure resin cement (Variolink II) was placed in a mold space of 5mm diameter and 0.75 mm thickness in between the ceramic and dentin disk. A silicone mold was prepared as the supporting structure of the dentin - resin cement - ceramic complex. During curing the temperature increase under the dentin was recorded using a J-type thermocouple.

It was concluded that

➤ Temperature increase varied significantly depending on the curing unit used.

➤ The plasma arc light unit caused significantly higher temperature changes compared to the other units ($3.7 \pm 0.2^{\circ}C$)

➤ The LED unit caused significantly lower temperature changes when compared to other units ($1.4 \pm 0.3^{\circ}C$)

➤ There was no statistically significant difference between the conventional halogen ($2.5 \pm 0.4^{\circ}C$) and high intensity halogen curing unit ($2.8 \pm 0.6^{\circ}C$)

➤ The maximum temperature increase determined was not viewed as critical for the pulpal health for any of the four curing units.

Danesh G et al[35] assessed and compared the temperature increase in the pulp chamber during resin based composite polymerization with two different light curing units, plasma arc lamp and conventional halogen light curing units. A class I cavity was prepared in an extracted lower molar such that remaining dentin layer was 1mm thick from the pulp chamber. The pulp chamber temperature rise was recorded for four different situations with two different curing units.

The light curing was done on

➤ The empty cavity

- ➤ Resin based composite only

- ➤ Resin based composite with cement base.

- ➤ Resin based composite with bonding agent.

The authors had concluded that

- ➤ The lowest temperature increase (0.3°C) was recorded during composite polymerization with a previously applied cement base using plasma arc lamp.

- ➤ The highest temperature increase (8.2°C) was recorded when using the conventional halogen light curing unit directly over the untreated cavity.

Kleverlaan CJ and de Gee AJ[36] had done a study to assess the curing efficiency of two fast halogen lamps (Astralis 10, Optilux 501) in three composites (Inten–s, Tetric ceram and Filtek Z 250) by measuring the hardness and depth of cure. They also determined the heat generated by these light sources. This study showed that the heat generation was less with Optilux 501 than Astralis 100 but there was no significant difference in curing efficiency between the two halogen lamps for the three resin composites. The temperature rise in the composites during curing was between 11.2°C and 16.2°C. The temperature rise during curing of each composite was significantly lower with the Optilux 501 than with Astralis 10. This was due to the spectral variation between the lamps as both have the same intensity.

3. MATERIALS AND METHODS

MATERIALS

1. Freshly extracted intact human mandibular molars

2. Dual cure Resin cements

   a. Relyx ARC (3M ESPE)

   b. Variolink II (Ivoclar Vivadent)

3. Resin Bonding Agents

   a. 3 M single bond adhesive (3M ESPE)

   b. Excite DSC (Ivoclar Vivadent)

4. Ceramic material (Vitadur alpha)

   a. core porcelain

   b. veneering material

5. Auto polymerizing acrylic resin

6. Silicon putty impression material

INSTRUMENTS AND EQUIPMENTS

1. Wheel diamond disc

2. Micro motor (kavo)

3. Micro motor hand piece

   a. Contra angle (NSK)

   b. Straight (NSK)

4. Digital Weighing machine (AND series HL – 200)

5. Metallic mold for ceramic disk preparation

6. Sagger tray

7. Digital Vernier caliper (Erskine Dental)

8. Light Curing units

    a. High intensity halogen (Heraeus Kulzer)

    b. Light emitting diode (Satelec)

    c. Light emitting diode (Mectron)

9. Stop clock

10. Ceramic furnace (Ivoclar Vivadent)

11. Digital thermometer (XMTG818-4071549)

12. K-type thermocouple sensor (Cr/Al)

13. Radiometer (Confident)

METHODOLOGY

A. Preparation of Dentin disks

Sixty teeth specimens (dentin disks) were prepared from extracted intact mandibular molars. Enamel portion from the occlusal surface of freshly extracted mandibular molars (free from debris, tissue tags and calculus) was removed to denude the dentin by trimming using a diamond wheel kept perpendicular to the long axis of the tooth. The same procedure was done on all other sides to obtain dentin disks of 10mm diameter. The disks were then fine trimmed to 1mm thickness using Arkansas stone. [*Figure 1*]

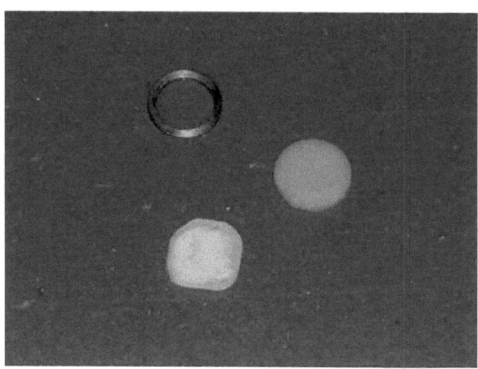

Figure 1: Ceramic and Dentin disk with Custom made Metal Ring Mold

B. Preparation of Ceramic Specimen

Ceramic disk was prepared with 2mm thickness and 10mm diameter. The disk was composed of 1mm thick framework material (core porcelain Vitadur alpha) and 1mm thick layering material [veneering material Vitadur alpha (dentine) EN2 A3 1053 LOT 7291]. To fabricate the ceramic disk, 0.2g of core porcelain powder was mixed with 3ml modeling liquid dispensed from a syringe. The mixture was placed in a metal mold of 1mm thickness and 10 mm diameter and condensed to get the desired dimension. The condensed material was separated from the mold and fired. Then the layering material was similarly weighed (0.2g) separately and mixed with modeling liquid (3ml). The mixture was placed in the metal mold and condensed to get the desired thickness of 1mm. The condensed material was separated from the mold and placed over the fired core porcelain specimen and was then fired together to get a 2mm thick 10mm diameter ceramic disk. [*Figure1*]

C. Experimental Set up

A round acrylic mold of 40mm diameter was created to support the silicone mold of 20mm diameter [*Figure2*].

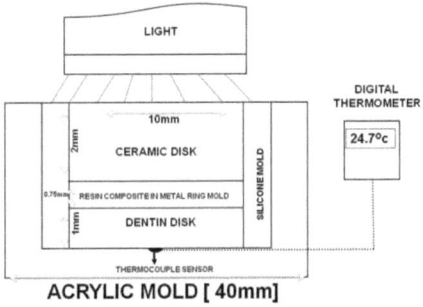

Figure 2: Experimental Set Up

The silicone mold in turn supported the dentin-ceramic disk complex[26]. The complex consisted of 2mm thick ceramic disk on a metal ring mold of 0.75mm thickness which rested on 1mm thick dentin disk. Therefore, silicone mold would be in contact with dentin disk followed by the dentin with metal ring mold, followed by the mold with ceramic disk [*Figure3*].

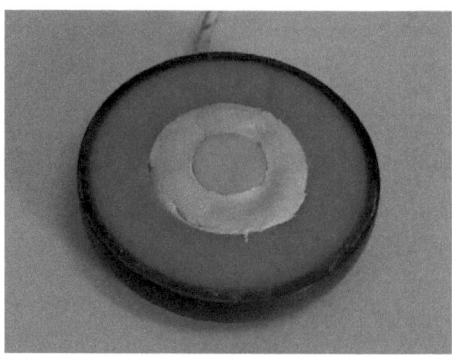

Figure 3: Specimen stabilized in silicone – acrylic complex

Presence of metal ring mold created space for resin luting cement. A K-type thermocouple sensor[20,29,34,36] wire was embedded in the middle of the acrylic mold so that the tip of the sensor contacted the dentin disk. The position of attachment was verified using radiograph[29,31] [*Figure 4*].

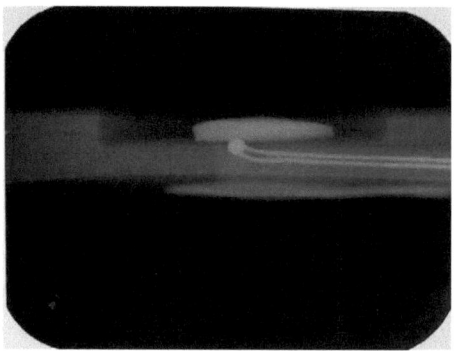

Figure 4: Contact of Dentin disk with sensor verified using radiograph

The temperature rise was recorded in the digital thermometer kept outside the complex.

Two commercially available dual cure resin cements (Relyx ARC, Variolink II [A$_3$ shade] - Table I) with their corresponding bonding agents (3M single bond adhesive, Excite DSC -Table II) and three different light sources (High intensity halogen with output of

$1060mW/cm^2$ - Heraeus Kulzer, LED with output of $1800mW/cm^2$ – Satelec, and LED with output of $800mW/cm^2$ Mectron - Table III) were selected for the present study.

Table I: Dual Cure Resin Cements used in the study

Brand name, Manufacturer	Lot no/ Shade	Filler particle size	Recommended curing time	Filler loading Wt. (%)
Relyx ARC 3M ESPE	FAFJ3415 /A3	1.5µm	40s in halogen	67.5%
Variolink II Ivoclar vivadent	BG28688 CG27068 /A3	0.7µm	40s in halogen	73%

Table II: Bonding agents used in the study

Brand name	Manufacturer	Lot no	Recommended curing time
3M single bond adhesive	3M ESPE	G51202	10s
Excite DSC	Ivoclar Vivadent	H23024	10s

Table III: Visible Light Curing Units used in the study

Brand, manufacturer	Type of unit	Output from light tip (mW/cm^2)	Diameter of tip (mm)	Duration of polymerization recommended by the manufacturer
Translux CL Heraeus Kulzer	High intensity halogen	1,060	8	40(s)
Mini LED, Satelec	Light emitting diode	1,800	7.5	20(s)
Starlight s, Mectron	Light emitting diode	800	8	20(s)

The bonding agents, resin cements and the light sources were combined to form twelve groups (Table IV).

Table IV: Distribution of Specimens

Groups	Curing light source	Sample description
Group I	High intensity halogen	3M single Bond adhesive Agent
Group II	High intensity halogen	3M single Bond adhesive + Relyx ARC resin Cement + Ceramic disk
Group III	High intensity halogen	Excite DSC Bonding Agent
Group IV	High intensity halogen	Excite DSC Bonding Agent + Variolink II resin Cement + Ceramic disk
Group V	Light emitting diode (Satelec)	3M single Bond adhesive Agent
Group VI	Light emitting diode (Satelec)	3M single Bond adhesive + Relyx ARC resin Cement + Ceramic disk
Group VII	Light emitting diode (Satelec)	Excite DSC Bonding Agent
Group VIII	Light emitting diode (Satelec)	Excite DSC Bonding Agent + Variolink II resin Cement + Ceramic disk
Group IX	Light emitting diode (Mectron)	3M single Bond adhesive Agent
Group X	Light emitting diode (Mectron)	3M single Bond adhesive + Relyx ARC resin Cement + Ceramic disk
Group XI	Light emitting diode (Mectron)	Excite DSC Bonding Agent
Group XII	Light emitting diode (Mectron)	Excite DSC Bonding Agent + Variolink II resin Cement + Ceramic disk

The light output of the curing units was measured to find out the level of intensity (>400 mW/cm^2 – necessary to cure the resin cement[27, 29]) before each experimental procedure using a digital curing radiometer under the ceramic – dentin complex.

D. Experiment and Temperature Measurement

Two coats of bonding agent were applied over the dentin disk. The light tip of the curing unit was cleaned, centered on the dentin disk and the bonding agent was cured for 10 seconds[1,37]. During curing of the bonding agent temperature was observed in a digital thermometer and recorded at every five seconds from the initiation of curing for two minutes (Figure 5).

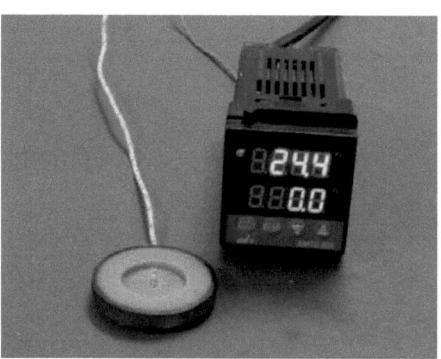

Figure 5: Thermocouple Sensor with Digital Thermometer

After sufficient cooling of specimens to room temperature of 25^{0}C, resin cement was mixed and placed over the cured bonding agent. Temperature of 25^{0}C was selected in accordance with the pilot study wherein we observed no statistical significant difference in temperature rise during irradiation, when the base temperature was 25^{0}C or 37^{0}C.

Dual cure resin cement was mixed in accordance with the manufacturer's instructions and then placed inside the 10mm diameter, 0.75mm thick metal ring mold, kept over the dentin disk. The ceramic disk was placed over this assembly and the curing of resin cement was done for the duration specified by manufacturer i.e., 40 seconds where high intensity halogen was used and 20 seconds where LEDs were used. Less time was used for LED since all of the spectral output of the LED was concentrated in the blue wavelength range[1,38].

The core portion of the ceramic disk was made to contact the dual cure resin cement. The light tip of the curing unit was centered on the ceramic restoration without any distance, to cure the dual cure resin cement. The temperatures were recorded every five seconds from the initiation of curing for two minutes. Total of 10 samples were assessed in each group.

The temperature rise was calculated between the initial and highest temperature for each sample (ΔT). The obtained reading (ΔT) was averaged for each group to determine the mean temperature rise for that particular group.

The results of the test were entered into an excel spread sheet (Microsoft) for calculation of descriptive statistics. Statistical analysis was performed using student's t-test and analysis of variance (ANOVA). Tukey's (HSD) tests were used to identify the significant pairs at 5 percent level (SPSS/PC, version 10.0, SPSS).

Research Design

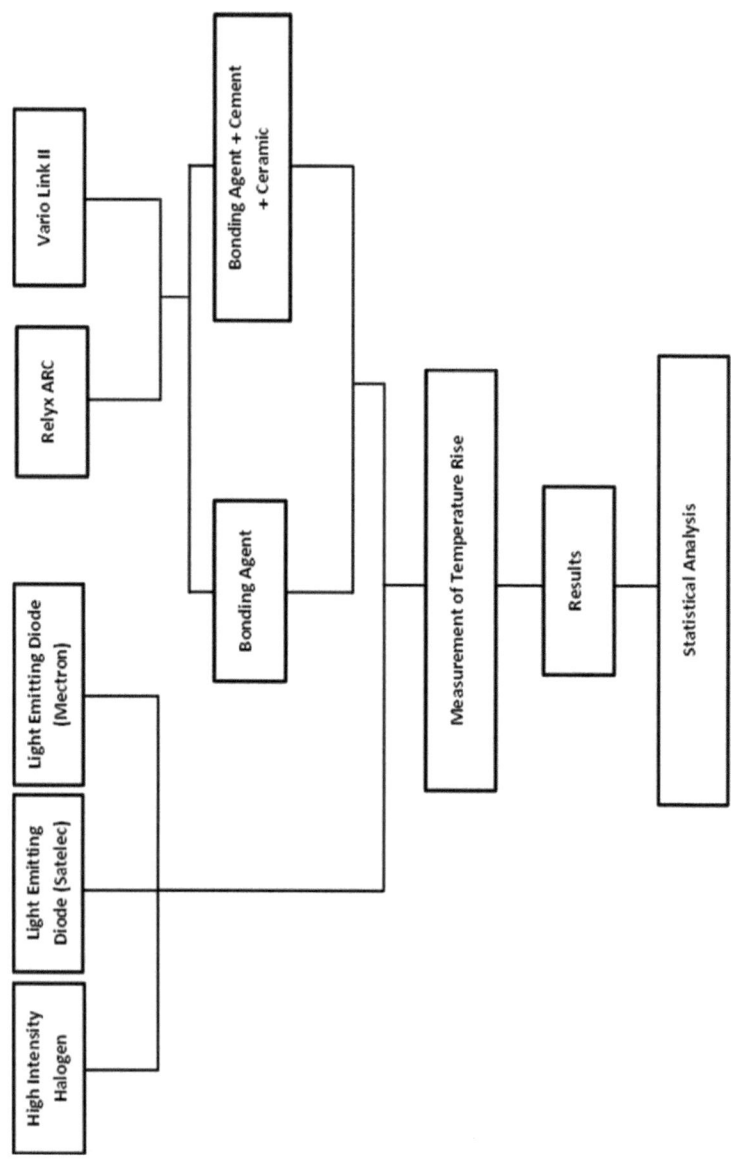

4. RESULTS

The mean rise in temperature by the different groups was summarized in the [**Table V**].

Table V: Mean rise in Temperature (ΔT ºC) for the Groups

Groups	Mean initial temperature (^{O}C)	Mean highest temperature (^{O}C)	Mean rise in temperature (^{O}C)	SD*
Group I	25.47	28.03	2.56	**± 0.41**
Group II	26.26	28.83	2.57	**± 0.21**
Group III	25.01	27.73	2.72	**± 0.46**
Group IV	26.16	28.89	2.73	**± 0.43**
Group V	26.6	29.77	3.17	**± 0.66**
Group VI	26.5	28.24	1.74	**± 0.32**
GroupVII	25.64	28.97	3.33	**± 0.43**
GroupVIII	26.47	28.38	1.91	**± 0.28**
Group IX	25.44	27.51	2.07	**± 0.25**
Group X	26.21	27.79	1.58	**±0.36**
Group XI	25.1	26.85	1.75	**± 0.36**
Group XII	25.87	27.25	1.38	**± 0.23**

*SD – standard deviation

The mean rise in temperature varied between 1.38°C and 3.3°C and varied according to the light curing unit, the dual cure resin cement and the bonding agent used. The lowest mean rise in temperature of 1.38°C was recorded when the dual cure resin cement Variolink II was cured using Mectron LED [Group XII]. The highest rise in temperature of 3.3°C was recorded when the bonding agent Excite DSC was cured using Satelec LED [Group VII].

When the comparison was made between different light curing sources for curing 3M bonding agent [**Table VI**],

Table VI: Mean, Standard Deviation and Test of Significance of Mean Values between two Bonding Agents under different Light Sources

Bonding Agents / Sources	3M single bond adhesive			Excite DSC		
	Groups	Mean (Std Dev)	*p value sig	Groups	Mean (Std Dev)	*p value sig
High intensity halogen	Group I	2.56 (± 0.414)	0.02 (s)	Group III	2.72 (± 0.461)	0.004(s)
Satelec [LED]	Group V	3.17 (± 0.660)	0.000(s)	Group VII	3.33 (± 0.435)	0.000(s)
Mectron [LED]	Group IX	2.07 (± 0.254)	0.07(n s)	Group XI	1.75 (± 0.362)	0.004(s)

[**Standard deviation in paranthesis, s-significant, ns-not significant, p-p value**]

Mean value of group **V** (3M single bond – Satelec) was higher than the mean value of group **I** (3M single bond – High intensity halogen) and **IX** (3M single bond – Mectron). There was a statistically significant difference in mean values between the group **V** and group **I** and **IX** at 5% level

When the comparison was made between different light curing sources for curing Exite DSC bonding agent [**Table –VI**], mean value of group **VII** (Excite DSC – Satelec) was higher than the mean value of group **III** (Excite DSC – High intensity halogen) and **XI** (Excite DSC – Mectron). There was a statistically significant difference in mean values among all the groups at 5% level

Under single light source for curing two different bonding agents the following results were observed [**Table –VI**].

a. Under High intensity halogen the mean rise in temperature during curing Excite DSC (Group **III**) was higher than the 3M single bond adhesive (Group **I**). However no statistically significant difference between the groups (Group **III** vs Group **I**) were found at 5% level.

b. Under LED Satelec the mean rise in temperature during curing Excite DSC (Group **VII**) was higher than the 3M single bond adhesive (Group **V**). However no statistically significant difference between the groups (Group **VII** vs Group **V**) were found at 5% level.

c. Under LED Mectron the mean rise in temperature during curing 3M single bond adhesive (Group **IX**) was higher than the Excite DSC (Group **XI**). Statistically significant difference between the groups (Group **VII** vs Group **V**) were found at 5% level.

The bar graph [Figure 6] shows that Satelec with Excite DSC produced highest temperature rise and Mectron with Excite DSC produced lowest temperature rise.

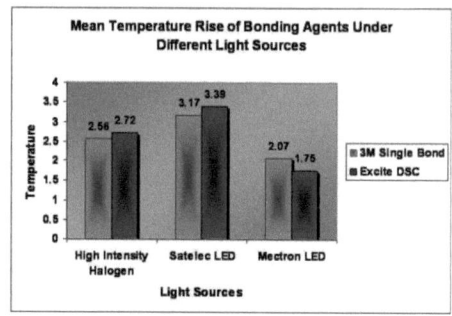

Figure 6: Mean Temperature Rise of Bonding Agents under Different Light Sources.

The graph [Figure 7] shows that Satelec LED group **V** produced highest temperature rise and Mectron LED group **IX** produced the lowest temperature rise. The temperature rise was steep and reached highest around 15 seconds.

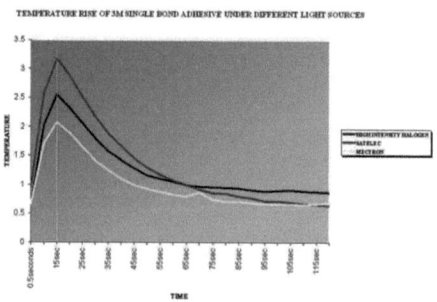

Figure 7 : Time Vs Temperature graph of 3M Single Bond Adhesive

The graph [Figure 8] shows that Satelec LED group **VII** produced highest temperature rise and Mectron LED group **XI** produced the lowest temperature rise. The temperature rise was steep and reached highest around 15 seconds.

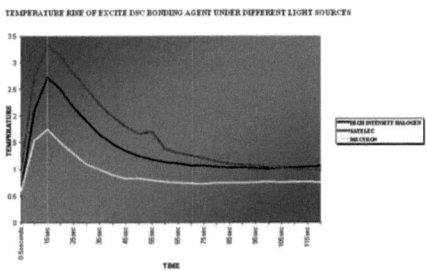

Figure 8: Time Vs Temperature Graph of Excite DSC

When the comparison was made between different light curing sources for curing Relyx ARC resin cement [**Table VII**],

Table VII: Mean, Standard Deviation and Test of Significance of Mean Values between two resin cements under different Light Sources

Resin cements / Light sources	Relyx ARC			Variolink II		
	Groups	Mean [Std Dev]	*p value sig	Groups	Mean [Std Dev]	*p value sig
High intensity halogen	Group II	2.57 (± 0.211)	0.000 (s)	Group IV	2.73 (± 0.432)	0.000(s)
Satelec [LED]	Group VI	1.74 (± 0.327)	0.488 (Ns)	Group VIII	1.91 (± 0.284)	0.003(s)
Mectron [LED]	Group X	1.58 (± 0.367)		Group XII	1.38 (± 0.234)	0.000(s)

[Standard deviation in paranthesis, s-significant, ns-not significant, p-p value]

Mean value of group **II** (Relyx ARC – High intensity halogen) was higher than the mean value of group **VI** (Relyx ARC – Satelec) and **X** (Relyx ARC – Mectron). There was a statistically significant difference in mean values between group **II** and group **VI** and **X** at 5% level

When the comparison was made between different light curing sources for curing Variolink II resin cement [**Table –VII**], Mean value of group **IV** (Variolink II – High intensity halogen) was higher than the mean values of group **VIII** (Variolink II – Satelec) and group **XII**

(Variolink II – Mectron). There was a statistically significant difference in mean values among all the groups at 5% level

Under single light source for curing two different resin cements the following results were observed [**Table –VII**].

a. Under High intensity halogen the mean rise in temperature during curing of Variolink II (group **IV**) was higher than the Relyx ARC (group **II**). However no statistically significant difference between the groups was found at 5% level.

b. Under LED Satelec the mean rise in temperature during curing of Variolink II (group **VIII**) was higher than the Relyx ARC (group **VI**). However no statistically significant difference between the groups was found at 5% level.

c. Under LED mectron the mean rise in temperature during curing of Relyx ARC (group **X**) was higher than the Variolink II (group **XII**). However no statistically significant difference between the groups was found at 5% level.

The bar graph [Figure 9] shows that High Intensity Halogen with Variolink II produced highest temperature rise and Mectron with Variolink II produced lowest temperature rise.

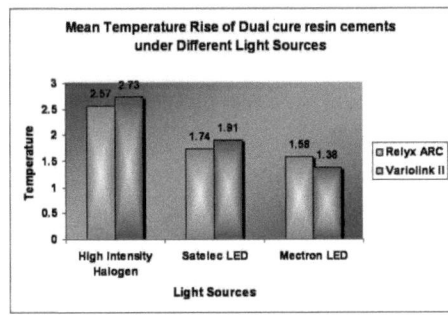

Figure 9: Mean Temperature Rise of Dual Cure Resin Cements under Different Light Sources

The graph [Figure 10] shows that High intensity halogen group **II** produced highest temperature rise and Mectron LED group **X** produced the lowest temperature rise. The temperature rise was shallow when compared to bonding agents and reached highest around 45 seconds.

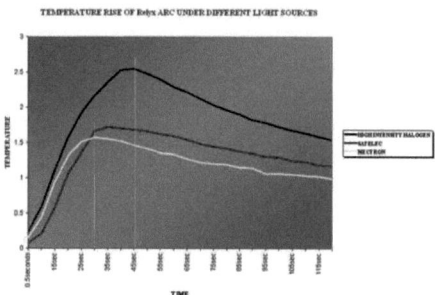

Figure 10: Time Vs Temperature graph of Relyx ARC under Different Light Sources

The graph [Figure 11] shows that High intensity halogen group **IV** produced highest temperature rise and Mectron LED group **XII** produced the lowest temperature rise. The temperature rise was shallow when compared to bonding agents and reached highest around 45 seconds.

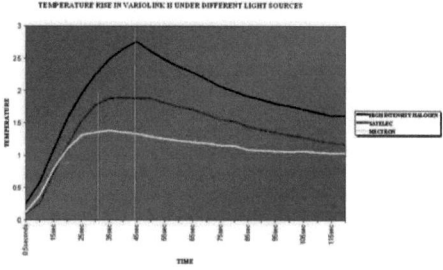

Figure 11: Time Vs Temperature graph of Variolink II under Different Light Sources

5. DISCUSSION

The damaging effect of temperature rise on pulp tissue during restorative treatment has been a matter of concern to dentistry for many years[20]. There is an evident thermal insult to the pulp from the light curing unit and from polymerization of the resin cement [21,28,36,39-41] while luting all ceramic restorations.

According to Lyod and Brown[17] and McCabe[16] light activation unit contributes greatly to the temperature rise and is more harmful than the restorative material. This temperature rise also depends on the type of curing unit[26,28,30,32,35,42] intensity of output[28,29] and irradiation time[28,29,42]. These factors should dictate the selection of light curing units.

The most commonly used curing units are high intensity halogen and light emitting diodes. LED lights used in this study has single peak since it uses single type of LED. LEDs produce a narrow spectrum of blue light because of its gallium nitride content in the 400- to 500-nm range (with a peak wavelength of about 460 nm), which closely matches the absorption spectrum of camphoroquinone (CQ), a photoinitiator widely used in light-activated dental resins[3,5,6,8-10]. It has been stated that LED LCUs polymerize more deeply than halogen lamps because they are more efficient on an equal energy basis[43].

Studies by Tjan et al and others[26,30,32] had showed that dentin thickness was a crucial factor in reducing the thermal transfer to the pulp. Our pilot study also showed that 1mm of dentin thickness was enough to reduce the temperature rise from 8-12°C to 1.3-3.5°C. Considering these factors the thickness and diameter of dentin disk (1mm thickness and 10mm diameter), ceramic disk (2mm thickness and

10mm diameter) and cement space (metallic steel mold of 0.75 thickness, 10mm external diameter and 8mm internal diameter to accommodate cement) were standardized.

Same dentin disks were used in earlier studies to eliminate the effect of histochemical and structural variables of teeth that may cause changes in thermal conductivity and specific heat[26,34]. In the present study due to curing of bonding agents the same dentin disk could not be used. To avoid bias, dentin disks were prepared and randomly selected.

A pilot study was conducted by us to determine the effect of environmental temperature on the temperature rise during irradiation using high intensity halogen with Relyx ARC. The experiment was conducted for the different environments (25°C and 37°C). Five readings were taken for both environments as the initial temperatures. The temperature rise was calculated and the results were analyzed using paired sample t-test. It showed that there was no statistically significant difference in the rise of temperature between the two initial environments. Hence the ambient room temperature of 25°C reported by Yap et al[20] was selected for the study.

The results of the present study showed that the LED (Satelec) registered the statistically higher mean temperature rise (3.17°C, 3.33°C) than high intensity halogen (Kulzer 2.56°C, 2.72°C) and LED (Mectron 2.07°C, 1.75°C Table: V). As the Curing time of bonding agents was kept the same for all the light sources, the output intensity [(LED Satelec 1800 mW/cm^2), (high intensity halogen Kulzer 1060 mW/cm^2), (LED Mectron 800 mW/cm^2)] might have played the key role.

The curing of resin cements gave a different scenario. Here the high intensity halogen (Kulzer 2.57°C, 2.73°C) registered the statistically higher mean temperature rise while curing the dual cure resin cements (Relyx ARC, Variolink II) as compared to LED units (Satelec 1.74°C, 1.91°C Mectron 1.58°C,1.38°C Table:V). This is in accordance with earlier studies[20,33,34]. The reason being curing time for dual cure resin cements is 40 seconds with high intensity halogen as per the manufacture's instruction[29,31]. LEDs cure the resin cements in 20 seconds which is half of the previous one. The lower thermal generation in LED is due to the lower irradiation time. Even though one of the LEDs light output intensity (Satelec 1800 mW/cm^2) was greater than high intensity halogen (1060 mW/cm^2) the curing time plays the major role here as it is almost half for the LEDs. Other causes

     a. use of hot filaments in high intensity halogen

     b. wider spectral output range[36] in high intensity halogen

Different LEDs varied significantly both in the curing of bonding agent[20] (Satelec {3M single bond 3.17°C, Excite DSC 3.33°C}, Mectron {3M single bond 2.07°C, Excite DSC 1.75°C} Table:V) as well as curing of resin cements (Satelec {Relyx ARC 1.74°C, Variolink II 1.91°C}, Mectron {Relyx ARC 1.58°C, Variolink II 1.38°C} Table:V). This is due to the fact that the output intensity varied significantly between them.

Under the same light source different dual cure resin cements and different bonding agents behaved similarly. This was due to the reason that magnitude of the exothermic reaction of the material does not contribute much to the temperature rise[30]. However it was observed that the bonding agents behaved differently only under the LED Mectron light (2.07°C 3M single bond, 1.75°C Excite DSC Table: V). The reason remains unexplained.

Pulp chamber temperature increase was measured continuously up to the point where the temperature begins to fall rather than the exact moment at which light curing unit was shut off. This was based on the pilot testing that showed the maximum temperature increase during the curing of bonding agent was at 5 seconds after the light curing unit was shut off. Sufficient useful data would be collected two minutes after the beginning of light curing. These findings were in agreement with earlier experiment[32].

It has been reported in the literature that 15% of the pulp failed to recover when the temperature rise in pulp chamber reaches 5.5°C (10°F) and 60% of the pulp failed to recover when the temperature rise in pulp chamber reaches 11°C (20°F)[25]. The highest temperature recorded (3.33°C Table: V) in the present study with various curing units, bonding agents and dual cure resin cements were well within the safety zone i.e., a rise that will not cause irreversible damage to the pulp.

The only limitation of the present study was that the temperature values measured here cannot be directly applied to temperature changes in vivo. The reason is that the experimental setup of this study did not consider heat conduction within the tooth during in situ curing of bonding agent and their corresponding dual cure resin cement. In a vital tooth the blood flow in the pulp chamber and fluid motion in dentinal tubules will probably show different rates of heating when exposed to curing lights. They may cool slower as well as heat faster. Temperature exceeding 43°C causes stimulation of efferent nerve fibers along with a reactive increase of blood circulation which dissipates the heat advancing toward the pulp chamber. In addition, the surrounding periodontal tissues could promote heat convection in vivo, limiting the intrapulpal temperature rise[29].

6. CONCLUSIONS

The conclusions drawn from the present in vitro study were

> ➤ Light sources have a significant influence on the rise of temperature in the pulp chamber of tooth during the curing of bonding agents and their corresponding dual cure resin cements.

> ➤ Choice of bonding agent does not cause a statistically significant difference in the temperature rise with the single light source (High intensity halogen and Satelec) except LED (Mectron) 3M single bond adhesive which showed the highest temperature rise.

> ➤ Choice of resin cement does not cause a statistically significant difference in the temperature rise with the single light source.

> ➤ The choice of LEDs (Mectron and Satelec) affects the temperature rise when curing the luting cements.

> ➤ Sufficient time interval of one minute should be given between curing of bonding agents and curing of their corresponding resin cements.

> ➤ The rise of temperature in all the groups may not affect the pulpal health as they were well within the critical temperature of $5.5^{\circ}C$.

REFERENCES

1. **Kramer N, Lohbauer U, Garcia-Godoy F, Frankenberger.** Light curing of resin based composites in the LED era. Am J Dent 2008;21:135-142.

2. **Stahl F, Ashworth SH, Jandt KD, Mills RW.** Light emitting diode [LED] polymerization of dental composites: Flexural properties and polymerization potential. Biomaterials 2000;21:1379-1385.

3. **Mills RW, Jandt KD, Ashworth SH.** Dental composite depth of cure with halogen and blue light emitting diode technology. Br Dent J 1999;186:388-391.

4. **Nakamura S, Mukai T, Senoh M.** Candela-class high brightness InGaN/AIGaN double heterostructure blue-light-emitting diodes. Appl Phys Lett 1994;64:16807-16813.

5. **Bouillaguet S, Caillot G, Forchelet J, Cattani-Lorente M, Wataha JC, Krejci I.** Thermal risks from LED and high-intensity QTH-curing units during polymerization of dental resins. J Biomed Mater Res Part B: Appl Biomater 2005; 72B: 260-267.

6. **Jandt KD, Mills RW, Blackwell GB, Ashworth SH.** Depth of cure and compressive strength of dental composites cured with blue light emitting diodes (LEDs). Dent Mater 2000; 16: 41-47.

7. **Oberholzer TG, Du Preez IC, Kidd M.** Effect of LED curing on the microleakage, shear bond strength and surface hardness of a resin-based composite restoration. Biomaterials 2005; 26: 3981-3986.

8. **Moon HJ, Lee YK, Lim BS, Kim CW.** Effects of various light curing methods on the leachability of uncured substances and hardness of a composite resin. J Oral Rehabil 2004; 31: 258-264.

9. **Awliya WY.** The influence of temperature on the efficacy of polymerization of composite resin. J Contemp Dent Pract 2007; 8: 9-16.

10. **Uhl A, Mills RW, Jandt KD.** Polymerization and light-induced heat of dental composites cured with LED and halogen technology. Biomaterials 2003; 24: 1809-1820.

11. **Price RBT, Felix CA, Andreou P.** Evaluation of a second-generation LED curing light. J Can Dent Assoc 2003; 69: 666-666i.

12. **Mills RW, Uhl A, Blackwell GB, Jandt KD.** High power light emitting diode (LED) arrays *versus* halogen light polymerization of oral biomaterials: Barcol hardness, compressive strength and radiometric properties. Biomaterials 2002; 23: 2955- 2963.

13. **Bennet AW, Watts DC.** Performance of two blue light-emitting-diode dental light curing units with distance and irradiation time. Dent. Mater 2004; 20: 72-79.

14. **Uhl A, Sigusch BW, Jandt KD.** Second generation LEDs for the polymerization of oral biomaterials. Dent Mater 2004; 20: 80-87.

15. **Haitz RH, Craford MG, Wiessman RH.** Handbook of Optics, Vol 2. New York: McGraw Hill, 1995:12.1-12.9.

16. **McCabe JF.** Cure performance of light-activated composites by differential thermal analysis (DTA). Dent Mater 1985;1:231-234.

17. **Lloyd CH, Joshi AE, McGlynn E.** Temperature rises produced by light sources and composites during curing. Dent Mater 1986;2:170-177.

18. **Masutani S, Setcos JC, Schnell RJ, Phillips RW.** Temperature rise during polymerization of visible light-activated composite resins. Dent Mater 1988; 4:174-178.

19. **Smail SRJ, Patterson CJW, McLundie AC, Strang R.** In vitro temperature rise during visible light curing of a lining material and a posterior composite. J Oral Rehabil 1988;15:361-366.

20. **Yap AUJ, Soh MS.** Thermal Emission by Different Light-Curing Units. Oper Dent 2003;28: 260-266.

21. **Dogan A, Hubbezoglu I, Dogan OM, Bolayir G, Demir H.** Temperature rise induced by various light curing units through human dentin. Dental Materials Journal 2009; 28(3): 253–260.

22. **Martins GR, Cavalcanti BN, Rode SM.** Increases in intrapulpal temperature during polymerization of composite resin. J Prosthet Dent 2006; 96: 328-331.

23. **Knezevic A, Tarle Z, Meniga A, Sutalo J, Pichler G.** Influence of light intensity from different curing units upon composite temperature rise. J Oral Rehabil 2005; 32: 362-367.

24. **Ozturk B, Ozturk AN, Usumez A, Usumez S, Özer F.** Temperature rise during adhesive and resin composite polymerization with various light curing sources. Oper Dent 2004; 29: 325-332.

25. **Zach L, Cohen G.** Pulp response to externally applied heat. Oral Surg Oral Med Oral Pathol 1965;19:515-530.

26. **Tjan AHL, Dunn JR.** Temperature rise produced by various visible light generators through dentinal barriers. J Prosthet Dent 1988;59:433-438.

27. **Barghi N, Berry T, Hatton C.** Evaluating intensity output of curing lights in private dental offices. JADA 1994;125:992-996.

28. **Shortall AC, Harrington E.** Temperature rise during polymerization of light activated resin composites. J oral rehabil 1998;25:908-913.

29. **Hanning M, Bott B**. In-vitro pulp chamber temperature rise during composite resin polymerization with various light curing sources. Dent mater 1999; 15: 275-281.

30. **Cobb DS, Dederich DN, Gardner TV.** In Vitro Temperature Change at the Dentin/Pulpal Interface by Using Conventional Visible Light Versus Argon Laser. Lasers Surg.Med 2000; 26: 386-397.

31. **Porko C, Hietala E-L.** Pulpal Temperature Change with Visible Light-Curing. Oper Dent 2001; 26: 181-185.

32. **Loney RW, Price RBT.** Temperature Transmission of High - Output Light Curing Units through Dentin. Oper Dent 2001; 26:516-520.

33. **Knezevic A, Tarle Z, Meniga A, Sutalo J, Pichler G, Ristic M.** Degree of conversion and temperature rise during polymerization of composite resin samples with blue diodes. J oral rehabil 2001; 28: 586-591.

34. **Usumez A, Ozturk N.** Temperature Increase during Resin Cement Polymerization under a Ceramic Restoration: Effect of Type of Curing Unit. Int J Prosthodont 2004; 17: 200-204.

35. **Danesh G, Davids H, Duda S, Kaup M, Ott K, Schafer E.** Temperature rise in the pulp chamber induced by a conventional halogen light–curing source and a plasma arc lamp. Am J dent 2004; 17: 203-208.

36. **Kleverlaan CJ, de Gee AJ.** Curing efficiency and heat generation of various resin composites cured with high intensity halogen lights. Eur J Oral Sci 2004; 112: 84-88.

37. **Mavropoulos A, Staudt CB, Kiliaridis S, Krejci I.** Light curing time reduction: in vitro evaluation of new intensive light-emitting

diode curing units. European journal of orthodontics 2005; 27: 408-412.

38. **Wiggins KM, Hartung M, Althoff O, Wastian C, Mitra SB.** Curing performance of a new-generation light-emitting diode dental cx uring unit. J Am Dent Assoc 2004;135;1471-1479

39. **Schneider LFJ, Consani S, Sinhoreti MAC, Sobrinho LC, Milan FM.** Temperature change and hardness with different resin composites and photo-activation methods. Oper Dent 2005; 30: 516-521.

40. **Al-Qudah AA, Mitchell CA, Biagioni PA, Hussey DL.** Effect of composite shade, increment thickness and curing light on temperature rise during photocuring. J Dent 2007; 35: 238-245.

41. **Hubbezoglu I, Dogan A, Dogan OM, Bolayir G, Bek B.** Effect of light curing modes and resin composites on temperature rise under human dentin: an *in vitro* study. Dent Mater J 2008; 27: 581-589.

42. **Goodis HE, White JM, Andrews J, Watanabe LG.** Measurement of temperature generated by visible-light-cure lamps in an in vitro model. Dent Mater 1989; 5: 230-234.

43. **Halvorson RH, Erickson RL, Davidson CL.** Polymerization efficiency of curing lamps: a universal energy conversion relationship predictive of conversion of resin-based composite. Oper Dent 2004; 29: 105-111.

ACKNOWLEDGEMENT

I hereby acknowledge Dr. Chandrasekaran Nair, Professor dept. of prosthodontics, Maruti dental college, Bangalore, and Dr.E.Munirathnam naidu professor and Director IDEA, Chennai, for their valuable suggestions during the course of my study.

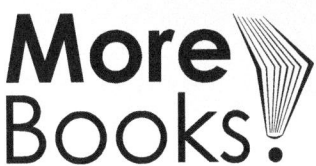

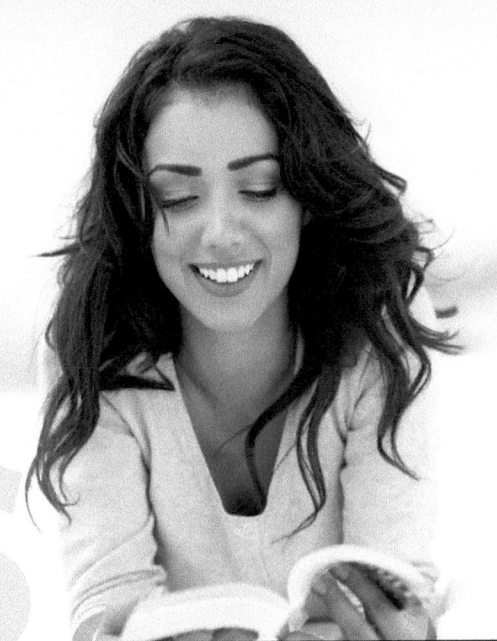

i want morebooks!

Buy your books fast and straightforward online - at one of world's
fastest growing online book stores! Environmentally sound due to
Print-on-Demand technologies.

Buy your books online at
www.get-morebooks.com

Kaufen Sie Ihre Bücher schnell und unkompliziert online – auf einer
der am schnellsten wachsenden Buchhandelsplattformen weltweit!
Dank Print-On-Demand umwelt- und ressourcenschonend produzi-
ert.

Bücher schneller online kaufen
www.morebooks.de

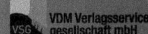 VDM Verlagsservicegesellschaft mbH
Heinrich-Böcking-Str. 6-8   Telefon: +49 681 3720 174   info@vdm-vsg.de
D - 66121 Saarbrücken   Telefax: +49 681 3720 1749   www.vdm-vsg.de

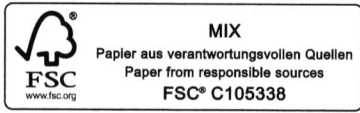

MIX
Papier aus verantwortungsvollen Quellen
Paper from responsible sources
FSC® C105338

Printed by Books on Demand GmbH, Norderstedt / Germany